Building a Trauma Kit

Gunner Morgan

Building a Trauma Kit

Reproduction or translation of any part of this work beyond that permitted by section 107 or 108 of the 1976 United States Copyright Act without permission of the copyright owner is unlawful. The author believes, to the best of his knowledge, that the information provide in this book is correct at the time of this writing. Requests for permission or further information should be addressed to the author.

DISCLAIMER AND/OR LEGAL NOTICES:

Care has been taken to confirm the accuracy of the information presented. However, the author and publisher are not responsible for errors or omissions or for any consequences from application of the information in this book and make no warranty, expressed or implied, with respect to the currency, completeness, or accuracy of the contents of the publication. Application of the information in a particular situation remains the responsibility of the practitioner.

Table of Contents

Trauma, Trauma Everywhere!

Think about the amount of time you spend stuck in traffic due to automobile accidents. There is rarely a day that I do not sit in traffic due to the congestion caused by a car crash. Police, fire, and ambulances block the roads making passage difficult. Then there are gawkers who have the compulsive need to slow down long enough to view the carnage hoping to catch a glimpse of ruin, destruction, devastation, and injury. Many don't want to look but they do anyway. It is human nature.

According to the World Health Organization[i]:

"Of all the systems with which people have to deal every day, road traffic systems are the most complex and the most dangerous. Worldwide, an estimated 1.2 million people are killed in road crashes each year and as many as 50 million are injured. Projections indicate that these figures will increase by about 65% over the next 20 years unless there is new commitment to prevention."

According to the U.S. Department of Health and Human Services[ii]:

"Motor vehicle-related deaths are a significant cause of preventable death, accounting for about

Building a Trauma Kit

35,000 deaths in the United States in 2010 across all ages."

How many parents have been fortunate enough to be spared a visit to the hospital emergency room for their kids cut, abrasions, or broken bones? Kids will be kids and it never fails that some of their mischievous behavior lands them in the emergency department for stitches or x-rays. For many kids it is a rite of passage. Getting that arm cast signed is a status symbol for some kids. Statistics from the World Health Organization state[iii]:

"Every day more than 2000 children die from an injury which could have been prevented."

Then there is the unpredictable world of violence and terrorism. America is no longer immune from terrorism and the world has been a violent place since the beginning of time. Rarely is there a news report that does not have some story about violence whether it be an assault, homicide, rape, bullying, gang violence, etc. It is a common sign of the times. Recently, the United States had the Boston Marathon bombing where pressure cookers were used to cause devastating injuries such as amputation of limbs. Additionally, active shooter situations have become common place such as Columbine, the Virginia Tech massacre, Sandy Hook, Aurora Movie Theater, Navy yard, etc. No location is immune from such violence.

Your workplace isn't much safer. Between 1997 and 2010, 79 percent of workplace homicides were shootings. Other homicides were the result of stabbing; hitting, kicking, and beating; assaults and violent acts by persons; and other means.[iv]

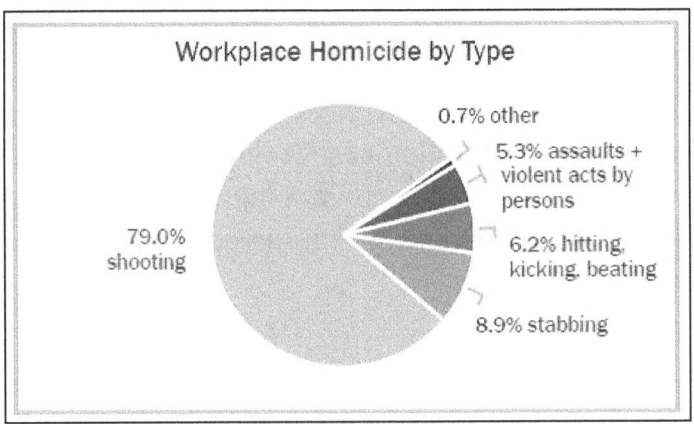

Natural disaster can be another cause of injuries that require immediate medical attention. Hurricanes, tornados, severe thunderstorms and flooding, wildfire, tsunamis, etc. can cause significant devastation. During the last few years the United States has experienced some major natural disasters that resulted in severe destruction, injuries, and loss of life.

According to the Annual Disaster Statistical Review 2012: The numbers and trends[v]:

"In the year 2012, natural disasters once again had a devastating impact on human society. Worldwide, 357 reported natural disasters caused the

death of more than 9,655 people, made 122.9 million victims and caused a record amount of US$ 157.3 billion of damages. A total of 120 countries were hit by these disasters. The five countries that were most often hit, China, the United States, the Philippines, Indonesia, and Afghanistan accounted for 38.1% of total disaster occurrence in 2012."

Living in a modern world means that we must be willing to accept the risks. There are a lot of methods that can cause severe injury requiring prompt medical attention. Trauma can result from the following:

- Accidents
- Violence
- Terrorism
- Workplace Violence
- Natural Disasters

No one is immune and injuries do not discriminate. Regardless of the source of injury it is a wise idea to be prepared to treat yourself or others. This requires obtaining first aid training, carry *quality* medical supplies, practice your skills, and attend ongoing training on a consistent basis. This is a huge responsibility that rewards you with the ability to save lives.

The focus of this book is going to be on developing a quality trauma kit that is capable of dealing with serious traumatic injuries from vehicular accidents, gunshot wounds, edged weapon attacks, falls, natural disasters and other sources. According to military research the two leading causes of death on the battlefield are from traumatic injuries are severe bleeding and chest wounds.

I will also provide suggestions for carry equipment for minor injuries as well. Traumatic injuries can range from big or small to minor or life-threatening.

Traumatic injuries can include the following:

- Cuts
- Avulsions
- Evisceration
- Amputation
- Penetrating injuries
- Blast injuries
- Blunt force trauma
- Deceleration injury
- Crush injury

Trauma can come from many different sources and the wounds can be devastating. Having a quality kit can be the difference between life and death.

DISCLAIMER:

The information provided is for educational purposes only. Do not provide care above your level of training. Neither the author nor publisher is responsible for how you use or misuse the information provided in this book. Seek appropriate medical training from a qualified source.

Do no harm.

Kit Priorities

Designing a trauma kit is a very personalized decision. It is impossible to cover all of the variables that go into designing a kit. For this reason, it is important for you to intimately know the reason for designing your kit. Additionally, there are many pre-packaged trauma kits on the market that go by a host of different names that can be modified to your requirements. It is up to you to design a trauma kit based upon your individual needs. Your priorities will depend on several factors that are unique to you such as:

- Your level of training
- Who you are willing to provide care to (self, family, others)
- How much money you are willing to spend
- How small or big you want the kit to be
- Weight considerations of your kit
- How often you are going to carry the kit
- Whether you are willing to replace used or expired components
- How long before a higher level of medical help arrives

Building a Trauma Kit

Your kit must be designed to handle the most severe case of trauma based on your level of training, skill, and experience.

The cost of a kit is a big factor for many people. I find that the best equipment typically comes with a higher price tag but you get what you pay for in terms of quality. My advice is to build a kit with the best quality components that you can afford. Even if this requires you to save up for some of the more expensive components it will be worth it to you and your patient. It has been my experience that cheaper quality components do not perform effectively which can be problematic when you are dealing with the worst case scenario. If you feel that it is taking you too long to save up for quality component think about how you would feel if you were treating a loved one with ineffective cheap medical gear! Sometimes we need to put things into perspective to stay on track.

Assessment

Answer the following questions as completely and honestly as you can. These questions will help you formulate the type of kit that will fit your needs or identify areas that you need to address.

1. What is your level of medical/first aid training?

_____None

_____Basic First Aid, CPR, CCR

_____Community Emergency Response Team

_____Emergency Medical Technician (EMT)

_____Paramedic

_____Military Training (Combat Life Saver, Medic)

_____Nurse

_____Physician Assistant

_____Doctor

_____Other: Explain: _____

_____

_____

Building a Trauma Kit

2. Who is your kit designed to treat?

_____Yourself (Self-aid)

_____Family - Friends

_____Anyone

3. How often are you going to carry the trauma kit with you?

_____Never

_____Rarely

_____Sometimes

_____Most of the time

_____Always

4. How are you going to carry the trauma kit?

_____Stored at home

_____On my person

_____In my vehicle

_____Stored at work

_____Other: _____

5. Specifically, what is your reason for designing a trauma kit?

_____

_____

_____

6. Are your kit components going to be:

_____Inexpensive (i.e., cheap)

_____Top of the line

7. Are you willing to replace old, expired, or used equipment?

_____Yes

_____No

8. Are you willing to attend refresher training or training to upgrade your current skills?

_____Yes

_____No

9. Are you familiar with the Good Samaritan Law in your respective area?

_____Yes

_____No

10. Do you live in an area that is:

_____Isolate

_____Rural

_____Suburban

_____Metropolitan

Answering these basic questions will provide you a starting point for designing your kit. The good news is that you can change your mind and go in a completely different direction if that suits your needs. The kit that you design will be uniquely your own creation based on your own needs. You have complete control on the design and implementation of your kit. Change it, modify it, and tweak it as you see fit.

Pre-Packaged Trauma Kits

You always have the option of purchasing a pre-packaged trauma kit but I tend to avoid going this route for a number of reasons.

It is my experience that premade kits:

1. Tend to cost more for what you are getting
2. Lack necessary components
3. Use poor quality components
4. Use less effective components
5. Sometimes come with components such as a hemostatic agent that is close to its expiration date
6. Are not designed for your individualized needs

Having said that, some kits are very comprehensive and high quality. The problem is that you may not know it until you get the chance to look at each individual component. You also have the option of buying a premade kit and adding quality components that fit your needs. I have purchased many kits over the years and I prefer to design a kit from scratch and build it based on quality components that fit my needs. If you are new to building kits this may mean that you have to conduct some testing and research which can be time consuming and expensive. For example, you might want to purchase an Israeli Dressing and a North American Rescue (NAR) Emergency Trauma Dressing to see which one you prefer. Both are excellent high quality products but your individual preferences may prefer one over the other. You may need to conduct tests on tourniquets, chest seals, bandages, etc. This may seem like a lot of work and it is. But it's important to remember that during an emergency is not the time to find out that you do not like the quality of the product. This is especially true if someone's life depends on the care that you are providing.

An excellent pre-packaged kit is the **Tactical Development Group Trauma Kit** by Rescue Essentials which retails for about $270.00 on Amazon.

The contents of this kit include the following:

> 1 - Maxpedition Fight Pouch (Kit Platform)
>
> 1 - Combat Application Tourniquet (C-A-T)
>
> 1 - SWAT-T Tourniquet
>
> 1 - Celox 35gm Packet
>
> 1 - Celox Trauma Gauze
>
> 1 - Bolin Chest Seal
>
> 1 - HyFin Chest Seal

1 - Nasopharyngeal Airway (28 fr) w/lube

1 - NAR Emergency Trauma Dressing, 6"

1 - NAR Emergency Trauma Dressing, 12"

2 - NAR S-rolled Compressed Gauze

1 - 7½" EMT Shears

1 - 12 Hour Light Stick

This kit will effectively treat the following:

Severe Hemorrhage: Utilizing Celox, CAT or SWAT-T tourniquet, trauma dressings, and compressed rolled gauze

Open Chest Wounds: Utilizing the Hyfin chest seal or the Bolin chest seal

Compromised Airway: Utilizing the nasopharyngeal airway

If you do not have the time or desire to conduct your own research on trauma kits this is a solid kit that can effectively handle severe trauma. On the downside there is no extra room in the kit to add any other supplies or individualize the kit to your needs. This kit is a bit bulky and will not fit in a pocket but can be used as a stand-alone kit with a shoulder strap, it can be placed in a backpack or attached using MOLLE webbing.

Building a Trauma Kit

There are smaller prepackaged kits available but remember that the smaller the kit the less it will have and there will be little to no redundancy. If you are a minimalist these kits may work well for you.

When designing a kit there is no right or wrong. There are only kits that have what you need in an emergency or they do not. You, as the designer of your kit, get to decide what your requirements are, the products that you carry, and how you are going to carry the kit. Whatever you decide is fine as long as it meets your needs. Do not feel pressured into purchasing components that you don't need, want, or do not have training to use. One of the best pieces of advice that I can offer is that you should take the time to think about your kit and the purpose it is going to serve.

Platform

The platform in which you plan on carrying your kit will be a significant factor in determining what you carry in your kit and how you carry your kit. Before choosing your platform I highly recommend that you first decide what components you are going to carry and then look at purchasing a platform that will effectively hold your gear. If you buy a platform first you may end up changing your kits components based on the limitations of the platform. This can dramatically impact your ability to provide effective emergency care.

If your plan is to carry a small kit in a pocket you are obviously going to be severely limited by size. It is very challenging to fit a comprehensive kit in a small package. If this is your plan it is then important to prioritize the purpose of your kit so that you know what components to include in the kit. If you are going to put your kit in a backpack, go bag, or everyday carry bag you have a lot more options for carrying a comprehensive kit. There are also some people who dedicate their whole backpack as a trauma kit. The problem I find with this set up is that you are only prepared for trauma/medical emergencies and nothing else. If you want to be well-rounded such as a prepper then I do not recommend dedicating a whole backpack to your trauma kit.

Building a Trauma Kit

Some of the smaller kits come vacuum sealed in a pouch that should not be opened prior to use. Others come in a carry case while others are part of a compartmentalized backpack that is a dedicated trauma/medical kit. Remember that the platform you use to hold your kit can be anything that fits your needs. Do not feel that you are obligated to use a specific type of platform. Use what works for you.

Some of the platforms that I have seen utilized include (some come fully stocked):

- Maxpedition FIGHT pouch
- Maxpedition FR-1 pouch
- Adventure Medical Kit (numerous versions)
- Variety of MOLLE pouches
- Elite First Aid Fully Stocked Rapid Response Trauma First Aid Bag
- First Aid Kit Emergency Response Trauma Bag Complete by My First Aid Company
- Ever Ready First Aid Fully Stocked First Responder Kit
- Condor Rip-Away EMT Pouch
- Medic Trauma Pack (CCRK) by North American Rescue - Price: $1,361.99
- Blackhawk Emergency Medic Roll Bag

- Blackhawk Omega Elite Modular Drop Leg Medical Pouch
- Blackhawk Special Operations Medical Backpack
- Voodoo Tactical Deluxe Professional Special Ops Field Medical Pack

As with the components of your kit I recommend that you use a high quality platform. This means that the platform material is durable for your needs, zippers are strong, webbing is strong, stitching is durable, and that the kit will stand up to abuse. The last thing you want to happen during an emergency is for it to have a catastrophic failure of your kit and have all of the contents fall out.

Trauma Kit

Below are items to consider when designing a trauma kit. While the focus of a trauma kit will be on trauma related injuries such as severe bleeding and open chest wounds I will also include items for problems that are not as severe. Even though the main priority is trauma it is important to have a well-rounded kit that is capable of handle minor trauma or medical conditions. You may decide to go strictly with a trauma kit. This is purely a personal preference. You are more likely to deal with minor injuries compared to major trauma. Again, design your kit based on your needs and level of training.

NOTE:

I am referring to the kit at a "*Trauma Kit*" but many different names are used such as FAK (First Aid Kit), IFAK (Individual First Aid Kit), etc. Do not get wrapped up in the minutia of a name. I could come up with a fancy name that sounds great but it is still a trauma kit. If you would like you may refer to your kit as a, "*High Speed Tactical Trauma Death Prevention Kit* or HST²DPK for short. It is just a name. You are better served by the components of your kit than the name you call your kit.

Following is a list of items that, in my opinion, are absolutely required components of a trauma kit:

- Tourniquet
- Hemostatic Agent
- Pressure Dressing
- Chest Seal
- Nasopharyngeal Airway (NPA)
- Gloves

I also believe in the concept of redundancy whereby I have multiple items that are the same or similar. The reason for this is because some products may break or be defective, you may need more than one, you may be treating multiple injuries, and you may be treating multiple people. When you carry redundant products it adds to the size, weight, and expense of your trauma kit. Again, this is a completely personal decision that you must decide. Keep in mind that things often break or go wrong at the worst possible time. Redundancy will help you get through these situations by being prepared for the inevitable problems that you encounter. Problems are the nature of the beast. Do not dwell on such problems during an emergency. Instead it is important to adapt, improvise, and overcome. Yes, it may sound cliché but it is the truth.

Critical Trauma Kit Components

⮑ Tourniquet

⮑ Hemostatic Agent

⮑ Pressure Dressing

⮑ Chest Seal

⮑ Nasopharyngeal Airway

⮑ Gloves

Tourniquet

A high quality commercially made tourniquet is one of the most important components of any medical kit. It is possible to bleed to death from an injury to a major artery in as little as 3-5 minutes. That is not a lot of time to address a severe hemorrhage. A high quality commercially produced tourniquet is essential.

According to the Journal of Emergency Medical Services[vi]:

"Recent military experience has overwhelmingly favored the efficacy of prehospital tourniquets. Their safety has been verified in routine use of tourniquets in the operating room and battlefield for the control of severe extremity hemorrhage."

The same article states a very important training point[vii]:

"Several important points need to be emphasized with regard to tourniquet training. The most important is that applying the tourniquet to the appropriate tension to achieve arterial occlusion can weaken the tourniquet. Microscopic tears develop in most commercial tourniquets using the dominant windlass mechanism necessary to achieve mechanical advantage. The package inserts for several tourniquets emphasize that tourniquets used

in training shouldn't then be used for actual treatment due to a much higher failure rate."

As this quote states it is critical to never train with the exact tourniquet that you are going to keep in your kit. Many companies now sell training tourniquets for this purpose. While this is yet another expense it is important for you to purchase a training tourniquet and not train with the tourniquet that is dedicated to your trauma kit.

I recommend the following tourniquets:

1. Combat Application Tourniquet   (C-A-T)

2. SOF Tactical Tourniquet (SOFTT)

3. Mechanical Advantage Tourniquet (MAT)

The reason that I recommend a high quality commercially produced tourniquet is because I do not want to improvise a tourniquet when someone is bleeding to death. If a person can die within 3-5 minutes from severe bleeding I want to use a tourniquet that is ready to go. I do not want to be searching my environment to see how I can improvise a tourniquet as the patient is bleeding to death. Having the ability to improvise is important but only when necessary.

Keep the following in mind when using a tourniquet:

- Tourniquets are to be applied approximately 2-3 inches above the wound
- Never place the tourniquet directly on the wound
- Tourniquets should not be placed directly over the knee or elbow
- The tourniquet can be placed over clothing if necessary but it is best if clothing is removed.
- Do not place a tourniquet over a cargo pocket that contains bulky items
- Once applied the distal pulse should be check to verify that the tourniquet is tight enough. If you still can feel a pulse then tighten the tourniquet more.
- A second tourniquet can be applied directly above the first tourniquet to control bleeding (This situation requires that you carry two tourniquets.)

Building a Trauma Kit

Common mistakes with tourniquet application include:

- Failure to apply a tourniquet when it is needed
- Waiting too long to apply the tourniquet which can lead to shock which can lead to death
- Failure to tighten it enough to eliminate the distal pulse
- Utilizing a tourniquet for minor bleeding
- Applying the tourniquet too high on the limb
- Removing the tourniquet prematurely

Using a tourniquet will often result in pain and discomfort which does not indicate that the tourniquet was incorrectly applied and it does not mean that it should be removed. Utilization of a tourniquet is necessary to save a life.

Hemostatic Agent

Hemostatic agents are used on bleeding where a tourniquet cannot be applied due to its location. There are many different types and brands of hemostatic agents currently available. A lot of research is being conducted on the development of new and more effective agents. This is an area to keep current on research and new products.

In the article *Prehospital topical hemostatic agents – A review of the current literature*[viii] it states:

"The perfect hemostatic dressing does not exist. Ideally, the dressing should be lightweight, easy to store, and able to be rapidly applied to a hemorrhaging wound. It should be conformable to the wound, allowing the hemostatic agent to reach areas of injury which are difficult to access with direct pressure (i.e. deep groin wounds). The dressing should cause minimal local tissue destruction, be easily removable from the wound, and not contain particles which can spread systemically. Finally, the dressing must not be washed away by rapid bleeding from high-flow blood vessels."

I recommend the following hemostatic agents:

1. QuikClot Combat Gauze
2. HemCon ChitoGauze Z-Fold by Chitogauze

Building a Trauma Kit

The two negative factors that many people complain about with hemostatic agents are that they are expensive and have an expiration date. It is true that a hemostatic agent will be one of the more expensive components in your kit. They typically have a shelf-life of about three years before needing to be replaced. The hemostatic agent that I use is QuikClot Combat Gauze.

Benefits of Combat Gauze include:

- Does not produce heat
- Highly effective in stopping bleeding
- Safe
- Conformable to wounds
- No known contraindications
- Three year shelf-life
- Simple and easy to use
- Product instructions are written directly on the package

When using a hemostatic agent such as QuikClot Combat Gauze it is critical to apply direct pressure for a minimum of three minutes.

According to the article previously mentioned[ix]:

"*Combat Gauze is a 3"x4 yard long roll of nonwoven gauze impregnated with kaolin. Combat Gauze has all the advantages of normal gauze (easy application, flexible, large coverage area, and easily removable) with the additional advantage of hemostatic function from the kaolin. It is designed for packing into deep wounds which are actively bleeding (i.e. arterial injury in the groin). Prehospital personnel can also use combat gauze as they would any standard Kerlix gauze. Combat Gauze was recently compared to several newer generation products, including the HemCon RTS, and found to be superior and had no apparent side effects. A study from the Israel Defense Force reviewed fourteen uses of Combat Gauze and noted a 79% success rate. The authors noted that in the three instances where Combat Gauze was unsuccessful, the soldiers had such severe injuries that only surgical control was successful. One of the three soldiers died from the severity of his wounds. Currently, Combat Gauze is the only product endorsed by the Tactical Combat Casualty Care Committee and they recommend it as first line treatment for life-threatening hemorrhage on external wounds not amendable to direct pressure and tourniquet placement.*"

Building a Trauma Kit

ChitoGauze Pro is another product that is becoming very popular and is touted as an excellent agent to stop bleeding. It is expensive at about $48.00. ChitoGauze Pro does not produce heat and offers antimicrobial properties against 26 bacterial organisms. In some recent medical studies ChitoGauze outperformed Combat Gauze. I may end up replacing Combat Gauze with ChitoGauze Pro after more research results are published. For now my go-to hemostatic agent will remain Combat Gauze.

Keep in mind that when using a hemostatic agent you may need to use more than one pack to effectively stop the bleeding. While this significantly adds to the cost of your kit it also significantly improves the chance that your patient will survive if you are effectively able to stop a severe bleed. You have to decide if spending the extra money is worth the expense when saving a life.

Pressure Dressing

Pressure dressings are applied on top of a hemostatic agent to assist with control of bleeding. The dressing must have the ability to exert pressure on the wound to be effective. They can also function as an improvised tourniquet, wrap, or sling to immobilize an appendage.

I use and like the following pressure dressings:

1. Emergency Trauma Dressing by North American Rescue (NAR)
2. Israeli Bandage

A lot of individuals express that they will use a tampon instead of a pressure dressing. I do NOT agree with this method for severe bleeding. A tampon is designed for bleeding due to a woman's menstrual cycle. This type of bleeding is significantly different than a severe arterial bleed that is spurting from a severed artery. In this situation a tampon will not effectively stop the bleeding. A tampon can be effective for a less significant bleed such as from venous bleeding due to an injury. The good news is that pressure dressings are not expensive.

Building a Trauma Kit

I utilize pressure dressings from North American Rescue called the Emergency Trauma Dressing (ETD) in both 4 and 6 inch. They also sell an Emergency Trauma Dressing Abdominal/Stump which is an oversized 12 in. x 12 in. sterile non-adherent pad. The ETD Abdominal/Stump is an excellent pressure dressing to treat traumatic amputations and abdominal eviscerations. An abdominal evisceration is where a section of intestine or other abdominal organ is displace through an open wound and protrudes outside of the abdominal cavity. Do NOT attempt to replace the protruding tissue back into the abdominal cavity. Keep in mind that medical training should be received for the proper treatment of abdominal eviscerations which is a severe injury that is extremely prone to infection. Carrying this pressure dressing will significantly add to the size of your kit as it is more bulky than the other pressure dressings.

All of the emergency trauma dressings are an effective sterile dressing used for applying direct pressure and have a shelf life of about 5 years.

Chest Seal

Rapid treatment of an open pneumothorax (sucking chest wound) consists of forming an occlusive seal over the wound which will help the patient breathe easier.

I recommend the following chest seals:

1. Hyfin Vent Chest Seal
2. Asherman Chest Seal
3. Bolin Chest Seal

According to new research published in the Journal of Special Operations Medicine[x]:

"All open and/or sucking chest wounds should be treated by immediately applying a vented chest seal to cover the defect. If a vented chest seal is not available, use a non-vented chest seal. Monitor the casualty for the potential development of a subsequent tension pneumothorax. If the casualty develops increasing hypoxia, respiratory distress, or hypotension and a tension pneumothorax is suspected, treat by burping or removing the dressing or by needle decompression."

I use the Hyfin Chest Vent Seal. This seal is a 6"x6" occlusive dressing used for the treatment of penetrating injuries to the chest.

When using a chest seal it is important:

1. To cover the wound during expiration (breathing out) with an occlusive dressing

2. That the occlusive dressing extends a minimum of two inches past the edge of the wound to provide the best seal possible

There are many commercially available chest seals available. Some of the more popular chest seals on the market:

- Hyfin
- Asherman
- Bolin
- Halo

The wound should be sealed on all four sides and the patient should then be placed in a sitting position if there are no other injuries. Application of an occlusive dressing should improve the patients breathing. The patient should then be monitored for the development of a tension pneumothorax which can result in increasingly difficulty breathing. If a tension pneumothorax develops the injured patient will need a needle decompression which needs to be performed by a person with appropriate medical training.

If there is a knife or other object impaled in the chest or other part of the body do not move the item or attempt to remove it. Leave in in place as the object may be controlling internal bleeding. If you remove the item it may cause internal bleeding that is difficult to control in the field. Attempt to secure the object with dressings for stabilization as best as possible so that it does not move and cause further injury.

Nasopharyngeal Airway (NPA)

A nasopharyngeal airway is used on a conscious, semi-conscious, or unconscious individual. One of the benefits of an NPA is that it is typically better tolerated by the patient than some other types of airways. The nasal airway typically does not cause the person to gag. NPAs should not be used on people with suspected head trauma or skull fracture. Use of an NPA typically requires formal medical training and should not be used without such training as there are some contraindications when using this airway. Improper use of an NPA can result in further injury.

I use the Rusch Nasopharyngeal Airway (28 Fr.) with Surgilube. Keep in mind that there are different size NPA's and there is no one universal size. The one that I carry is not meant to be used on a child because it would be too large.

Insertion of a Nasopharyngeal Airway is not a difficult skill yet it is still best that you receive appropriate hands on training from a qualified medical provider in its application. It is also important to know that there are some contraindications for using a NPA which will be covered in training.

NPA's are inexpensive typically costing less than $8.00 for a high quality product.

Gloves

Gloves are an essential piece of protective equipment and must be worn whenever treating another person to provide protection from bloodborne pathogens such as hepatitis, HIV/AIDS, and others. Bloodborne pathogens are viruses, bacteria and other micro-organisms that:

- Are carried in a person's bloodstream
- Cause disease

Always wear gloves when working around all body fluids and keep in mind that there are other body fluids besides blood which can contain pathogens. Due to the nature of traumatic injuries it is possible to encounter peritoneal fluid, cerebrospinal fluid, synovial fluid, pleural fluid, pericardial fluid, vomit/feces, saliva, and amniotic fluid. Just because a fluid is not the color red does not mean that it is not infectious. Always protect yourself. Exposure can occur in three ways:

1. **Direct Contact** – Direct physical transfer between a susceptible host and an infected individual

2. **Indirect Contact** - Personal contact with contaminated objects such as used door knobs, instruments, soiled clothes, etc.

3. **Droplet Contact** - Projection of a droplet sprayed onto a person as a result of sneezing or coughing. You should also consider a face mask and/or goggles. Such protective equipment will protect you from breathing in droplets or having them hit your eye.

Bloodborne pathogens cannot pass through intact skin but they can enter the body through:

- Abrasions
- Acne
- Blisters
- Burns
- Cuts
- Mucous membranes - eye, nose & mouth
- Open sores
- Punctures from needles or other sharps

I use Black Talon Nitrile Gloves because they fit well, are hypoallergenic, durable, and still allow for good sensation when taking a pulse, inserting an I.V. or performing a needle decompression. If you live in a warm climate it is not a good idea to leave gloves in your hot vehicle as the heat will degrade the gloves rendering them ineffective. I recommend that you replace your gloves on an annual basis if they are exposed to heat.

Bloodborne Pathogens

Are viruses, bacteria, and other micro-organisms that:

➲ **Are carried in a person's bloodstream**

➲ **Cause disease**

Always Use Protective Gloves

Bloodborne pathogens *CANNOT* pass through intact skin

But they <u>can</u> enter the body through:

➲ Abrasions
➲ Acne
➲ Blisters
➲ Burns
➲ Cuts
➲ Open sores
➲ Mucous membranes - eye, nose & mouth
➲ Punctures from needles or other sharps

Building a Trauma Kit

Additional Components

The contents listed above are effective for handling major trauma. But, not all accidents and injuries are major. In fact, the majority of what you will encounter, depending on your profession and activities, will probably be relatively minor. Also, the majority of people live in an urban environment where quality medical and emergency care is readily available. Therefore, it is always a good idea to have other items in your kit for less serious injuries. This will provide you with a well-rounded kit that is highly capable especially if you live a long way from medical care, are on an outing in the wilderness, are out hunting, or maybe you are a prepper who wants a versatile kit. Also, there are people who have multiple medical kits depending on their needs. For example, they may have a trauma kit, medical kit, vehicle kit, home kit, individual kit, hunting kit, etc. These kits are all geared toward a specific purpose. You may choose to go this route.

There are some items that I feel everyone should carry all of the time that are not necessarily part of a medical/trauma kit but have a lot of value. These items are often referred to as everyday carry or EDC. I am not going to go over every possible EDC item just a few that will complement an emergency medical kit.

Items to complement a medical/trauma kit:

- **Flashlight** – The flashlight does not have to be large or too powerful. The idea is to have a light that you are capable of seeing your equipment in a low light situation. I use the Streamlight 88032 Protac Tactical Flashlight 1AA. I like that it uses one inexpensive and easy to find AA battery compared to a CR123A battery. The light output is 110 lumens on the high setting and 12 lumens on the low setting. Be sure to always carry a spare battery with you. I also change my battery every January 1st regardless of how old the battery is so that I know I start off the New Year with fresh batteries in all of my equipment. There are many excellent flashlights to choose from so find one that meets your needs. Do NOT use this light on high output to check for a pupillary response.

- **Knife** – A good quality knife is always a useful instrument to carry. For the purposes of your kit you do not need a huge hunting, tactical, or bushcraft knife. A small Swiss Army knife will work fine. This knife will be used to cut clothes if necessary or open items. The key is to make sure the knife is sharp and I recommend a locking blade. An excellent and simple knife is the Victorinox Swiss Army One Hand Sentinel Pocket Knife. All it has is one blade that locks. If you want to carry a little bit more you can also look at the Victorinox Swiss Army One-Hand Trekker

Lockblade Pocket Knife. You have a lot of choices when it comes to knives.

- **Watch** – Chances are you already wear a watch so this will not be a big change for most people. The watch should have a second hand or show seconds if it is digital. The reason for this is so that you can monitor a patients pulse and respirations. Vital signs can provide significant information on a patient's condition such as whether they are deteriorating or stabilizing. I use a Timex Expedition. It isn't fancy but it gets the job done.

- **Pen and Pad** – This does not have to be anything spectacular, big, or expensive. A pen and pad is useful for writing down important information that you may forget. For example, you are a long way from help you may be with a patient for an extended period of time. It is a smart idea to write down information such as the time you arrived or the time the accident happened, keep track of vital signs to develop a trend, note the time a tourniquet was applied, or gather relevant patient information in case the person loses consciousness. It is especially important to obtain information on all allergies, medications the person is taking, and current medical conditions. This information can then be provided to whoever takes over medical care. I use a Rite in the Rain

All Weather Pocket Notebooks that is 3" x 5" with a weatherproof pen.

The items listed above are very valuable when dealing with medical or trauma issues. The items should not be problematic to implement into the set up that you design. Their utility will be invaluable should you need those items during an emergency. In an emergency you are not going to remember everything so having a pen and pad to document important items should not be overlooked or underestimated in its value.

From here we are working under the assumption that you are looking for a more comprehensive kit for medical and trauma related emergencies *and* non-emergencies. I want to stress that you do NOT need to carry every item that I am going to list. If you do you may end up with a huge complicated kit. I am also not going to list every single possible item that you could carry. This is why it is so important to figure out what you need for your specific situation. You may decide to go with a very small and minimal trauma kit, one huge comprehensive kit, or break your kit down into multiple, or what I call modular, units. There is no wrong answer as long as the kit meets your needs.

Building a Trauma Kit

<u>Additional items to consider for your kit:</u>

- **EMT Shears** – These shears are great because they can cut through just about anything including thick leather boots and jackets. The person you cut them off may not be very happy with you if you cut through their favorite shirt, pants, or boots so just remind them that you are there to help. It is always a good idea to communicate with your patient to let them know what you are going to do before you do it and tell them why you are doing it. In a true emergency do not take the time to do this and instead focus on providing excellent patient care. Not all EMT shears are made equally so do some research and buy a quality pair. They are very handy to have available.

- **SurgiPad** – I like to use the Johnson & Johnson Red Cross Surgipad Surgical Dressings, 5 Inch x 9 Inch. These are large thick pads that work well for larger cuts.

- **Mylar Space Blanket** – These work well for prevention of hypothermia, maintaining body temperature, and providing privacy if needed. They are very small and inexpensive. I keep Mylar Space Blankets in each of my kits. I use the Adventure Medical Kits Sol Survival Blanket.

- **Assortment of Bandages and Tape** – There are so many different types and sizes of bandages available that it can get confusing. Do not get too wrapped up in all of the choices. Remember, larger bandages can be cut down in size to make smaller bandages. I like to carry an assortment of different bandages such as All-purpose Sterile Sponge 4" X 4", eye patch, and varying sizes of Band-Aids and butterfly closures. I also use self-adhesive roll tape to keep bandages in place along with a self-adhering ACE bandage.

- **Triangular Bandage** – The great thing about a triangular bandage is that it is so versatile and can be used for many tasks such as securing an arm in place, making a sling, improvising a tourniquet, using it to hold a dressing in place, etc. Also carry some safety pins. I carry 3 large safety pins and 3 small ones.

- **Burn Gel** – If you have ever experienced even a minor burn you know it can be extremely painful. Hands down the best product I have used for burns is Water Jel Burn Jel which comes in different formats. I like the 1/8 ounce packets for smaller burns and Water Jel Burn Dressing, which come in an assortment of different sizes, for larger burns. These products help to rapidly cool the burn to prevent further damage. All burns should be treated by a medical professional due to the high risk of infection and complications from burns such as scarring.

Building a Trauma Kit

According to the Water-Jel Technologies website[xi]:

"When a burn occurs, seconds count. Water-Jel products are effective, versatile and approved for emergency first aid burn treatment in a pre-hospital setting. Water-Jel products are consistent with both wet and dry burn treatment protocols since they stop the burning process, cool the burned area, relieve pain, prevent further injury and do not contribute to hypothermia or interfere with debridement (removal of damaged tissue or foreign objects from a wound). There are no active ingredients, and the water-soluble gel can be easily washed off at a hospital or burn center.

Water-Jel is scientifically designed to draw the heat out of a burn. The heat energy is spread over the whole gel surface because the material conforms to the uneven burn surface. At the outer surface of the gel, the heat is released by transfer into the air. The buffer effect of the Water-Jel layer leads to rapid heat transfer out of the burn wound without losing temperature around the area of usage."

I have used this product on a few occasions on first and second degree burns and it worked very effectively in stopping the pain.

- **<u>Antiseptic Sanitizer</u>** – With all injuries infection is always a serious concern and can lead to death if not treated. It would be very unfortunate to survive the trauma to die from an infection. One option to use Betadine Swab Aid Antiseptic Pads because they are easy to carry. The problem is that the swab can dry out over time. Another option is to carry a small bottle of Betadine but the tradeoff is that it is bigger and bulkier. I also carry either a small tube or small packets of triple antibiotic ointment. I like the ointment because it stays on better than cream. These products are good when dealing with smaller wounds.

  A small 1 ounce bottle of hand sanitizer is also a good idea so that you can clean your hands before and after treating a patient. Even when you use hand sanitizer after treating a patient it is good practice to wash your hands with soap and water as soon as possible. Hand sanitizers should be used as a "temporary" solution until you can wash with soap and water.

- **<u>Sam Splint</u>** – This splint is great because it is so versatile and malleable for many uses from splinting a broken bone to providing stability to a potential neck injury. They now come flat or in a roll so you can choose the one that will best fit into your kit. They come in bright orange or subdued olive green.

- **<u>Tweezers and Hemostat</u>** – Tweezers are an invaluable item for those times you get something stuck in your skin. Do not skimp and buy a cheap pair. Many pocket knives come with small tweezers that are virtually useless and have no grip. Good tweezers are a must and this is one of those items that I carry two. In conjunction with tweezers get a good quality magnifying glass. Years ago I was hiking in the desert and ran into a family with a small boy of about 5 years old. He was resting on a rock and when he went to get up he inadvertently put his hand on a cactus and had over 100 cactus needles in his hand. Fortunately, I had my tweezers and about a half hour later we were all on our way. A tough lesson learned for that young boy.

  A hemostat is a multifunctional item that can be used to clamp items especially an artery that is spurting blood. Most people might not be willing to do such a drastic maneuver but it is an option.

- **<u>Mole Skin</u>** – This is one of those products you rarely give thought to until you start developing a painful blister. It is small and worth having in your kit especially if you are backpacking in a remote area. Remember, when in the remote outdoors it is critical to take care of your feet.

- **Duct Tape** – Everyone knows that there are so many uses for duct tape that it is a no brainer to keep some in your kit. I find that Gorilla Brand duct tape is one of the best on the market and I keep this in all of my kits. Duct tape is versatile and allows you to improvise on the spot.

- **CPR Mask** – The reality is that many patients vomit when CPR is performed. Having a mask will provide you a layer of protection. I recommend the Laerdal Pocket Mask which can be used on adults, children, and infants.

- **Face Mask and Goggles** – When we discuss the use of gloves, face mask, and goggles we are really discussing the concept of utilizing personal protective equipment (PPE) which protect you from becoming infected from bloodborne and airborne pathogens.

  A face mask will help in preventing you from inhaling airborne pathogens such as tuberculosis. They are also good to use as a form of protection when treating people who may have been exposed to the flu or other virus.

  Goggles will also function well in an environment that is full of dust or debris. Do not underestimate the importance of protecting your eyes. You will become very ineffective if you lose the ability to see.

- **Headlamp** – This is one of those items that come in very handy when dealing with a trauma or medical condition in a low-light situation. You do not want to have to hold a flashlight in your hands and I do not recommend putting it in your mouth. Always avoid placing items in your mouth especially because they may have become contaminated. A headlamp will allow you to avoid this situation and provides you the ability to use both of your hands.

- **Needle for Chest Decompression**

  NOTE: A chest decompression must only be used by individuals who are trained and authorized in this procedure.

  This product is used to treat a tension pneumothorax which is a life-threatening condition. I recommend the ARS for Needle Decompression (14 gauge x 3.25 in) which is sold by North American Rescue for $9.99 and requires medical device authorization to purchase. This is a small, compact, and inexpensive piece of equipment that can truly save a life in the hands of a trained individual. Continuing your medical education to obtain this valuable skill is very valuable.

Medications – Over the Counter and Prescription

It is important to note that over the counter medication and prescription medications are not harmless and can cause serious problems to include death. I do not advocate giving over the counter medications to another person outside of your family except in certain circumstances. The reason is because you do not know if the person has an allergy to the medication or if it will negatively interact with current medications that the person is taking. I would never give an over the counter medication to a child that is not mine. I might provide it to the child's parent(s) and then let them make the decision to give it to their child.

NEVER give your prescription medication to another person as this violates state and federal law and can lead to criminal charges. If you take a pill that was prescribed to someone else or give that pill to another person, it is not only potentially harmful, it is illegal.

But, you probably want to have some medications available for yourself and your family. Make sure that each family member knows what each medication in your kit is for, who it is for, and the correct dosage. This is especially important if something happens to you. This is also a good reason to make sure that all medication, prescription and non-prescription, are properly labeled. Additionally, many medications are labeled to keep medicines in a cool, dry, secure place out of a child's reach. Many medications are also susceptible to heat, air, light, and moisture. These factors make storing your medication in your kit very problematic.

- **Prescription Medication**

  Legally, all prescription medication that you carry is supposed to be in the prescription bottle that you received it with the label attached. It is also important to make sure that the method you carry the medication does not degrade it such as exposing some medications to heat or light. This can be challenging when placed in your kit especially if it is stored in your vehicle. If you decide to carry your medication in a different location than your prescription bottle it is critical to clearly and accurately write the prescription information on the container. Do not go by memory because you may not be thinking clearly in an emergency especially if it is you that is hurt or sick. I recommend carrying a three day supply of each medication that you and your family members take in case you are in a situation where you are delayed in getting to appropriate medical care. You may choose to carry a supply that is longer than 3 days. A good method to obtain some extra medication is to ask your physician for samples when you have an appointment. This will not work for all medications such as narcotics.

Prescription medication you may choose to carry that you do NOT regularly require (These medications are for those just in case scenarios):

- ⮑ Pain Medication – Percocet, Vicodin
- ⮑ Muscle Relaxer – Soma, Flexeril
- ⮑ Nausea/Vomiting - Promethazine (Phenergan)
- ⮑ Anti-Anxiety – Xanax, Ativan
- ⮑ Antibiotic – Broad Spectrum
- ⮑ Allergy – Auto-injectable epinephrine which is used to treat a life-threatening allergic reaction known as anaphylaxis from insect stings. Fluticasone propionate, Levocetirizine, etc.

Think twice **BEFORE** taking a prescription medication even if you have taken them previously in the past. The reason is that there are many side effects you may experience which are not beneficial during an emergency. Many of the medications listed above can cause sleepiness and drowsiness. If you need to remain alert and focused these medications can impair your ability to do so. You might need to deal with some pain and discomfort.

Unless your physician says otherwise, if you are in a situation where medical assistance is on the way to your location I do NOT recommend using prescription medication. Paramedics or the hospital will provide you with medications that you require. If you are having chest pain due to a possible heart attack, which is a medical condition, your doctor may have prescribed nitroglycerin tablets for you to take prior to the arrival of first responders. Always follow the advice of your medical provider.

On the other hand, if you are in a situation where you receive an injury and help is going to be *delayed*, such as on a backpacking trip, a major natural disaster, or breakdown of society consider using the medication to alleviate your symptoms. This may work well if you are not alone and there is at least one person who can look after you. If help is not coming and you are going to have to get to safety on your own then resorting to pain medication or muscle relaxers might be your only option. Keep in mind that the side effects may make you tired and can lead to poor decision making. In such cases use extreme caution so that you do not cause further injury.

When dealing with prescription and over the counter medications it is important to know the pros and cons of consuming the medication. Every medication has potential side effects and different individuals can respond differently to the same medication. Do not assume that because you tolerate a medication well that someone else will have the same experience. For example, some people can take Benadryl (Diphenhydramine) which is an over the counter medication and function well while others will become extremely tired and need to sleep.

- **Over the Counter Medication**

  These readily available medications are so common place that we forget that they can be dangerous. Make sure that you understand and know the indications, contraindications, possible side effects, and dosages before using any of these medications. It is also important to know if these medications interact with prescription medications, herbal supplements, or vitamins that you are currently taking.

  Over the counter medication you may choose to carry (Remember, you do not have to carry any or all of these):

  - Anti-inflammatory and/or fever reducer – Aspirin – Heart attack (Do not give aspirin to children), Tylenol, Advil, Naproxin
  - Anti-Diarrheal – Lotrimin AD
  - Anti-Histamine – Benadryl, Zyrtec, Sudafed, Cortisone ointment
  - Antacid – Tums, Prevacid, Tagamet, etc.
  - Eye Drops – Clear Eyes, Similasan Dry Eye Relief, Systane Ultra Lubricant Eye Drops, etc.

- ⮥ Cough Medicine – Cough drops (Halls), Mucinex, Dextromethorphan, Guaifenesin, etc.
- ⮥ Antibiotic – Triple Antibiotic ointment
- ⮥ Other: Vaseline Lip Therapy, Sun Block, Lotion, anti-bacterial wipes

▪ **<u>Medical Alert Tag & List of Medications</u>**

Keep in mind that you may end up being the patient. If you have any medical conditions or allergies it is very important to have a medical alert tag or medical ID tag documenting this information. It can be a necklace, bracelet, or placed in your wallet.

It is also important to keep an up to date list of all medications that you are taking along with the name of the medication, dosage, how often you take the medication, and your doctor's name and phone number. On this list also include any supplements that you take such as vitamins and herbal medicine. A good technique to ensure that this information is found by first responders is to use a paper clip and attach your medication list to your driver's license or identification card if you do not drive.

Medical Alert Tag

Especially important when you are the patient!

Allergies:

Codeine & Sulfur

Dexter Warner

DOB: 05-29-1984

Emergency Contact: 212-555-1234

Wound Suturing

Lately there has been a fad of sorts on suturing wounds. This has become a very popular topic with an explosion of available resources. There are videos, blogs, webpages, and even seminars on this skill. While I believe training in medical skills is important I am not supportive of suturing wounds as my **primary** course of action as there can be significant complications associated with using incorrect technique and procedure. I am not against learning this skill and encourage you to do so but use this information responsibly. This means that you should have everything you need available to effectively suture the wound while minimizing further problems or complications. Wounds come in many different forms such as simple lacerations, skin avulsions, very deep wounds, crush injuries, amputations, etc. Wounds can be clean, contaminated, or infected. You may not have medicine such as Lidocaine to anesthetize the wound. If you do not have access to an anesthetic for pain then suturing is going to hurt.

Chances are that any specialty class or seminar that you attend will provide very basic information on simple lacerations but not cover all variables. If you do not know what you are doing you may end up causing more harm that will need to be addressed at a later time by a qualified medical professional. Complications from incorrect laceration repair include scarring, retained foreign body, to a life-threatening infection that potentially kills the patient.

If you are committed to learning how to suture keep the following in mind:

- Suturing should be your **_last_** resort to close a wound
- There are alternative options to close a wound such as:
  - ⇒ Band-Aid
  - ⇒ Gauze dressing and tape
  - ⇒ Steri-strip / Butterfly tape
  - ⇒ Glue
- Before you attempt to close the wound you must stop the bleeding
- Attempt to clean the wound as good as possible
  - ⇒ Wash your hands prior to working on the patient
  - ⇒ Always wear protective gloves
  - ⇒ Use water to irrigate the wound
  - ⇒ Use an irrigating syringe to flush dirt and debris from the wound
- Do not use hydrogen peroxide as it is cytotoxic meaning that it will kill cells which impairs and delays the healing process while increasing the risk of infection
- If you use betadine for dirty wounds you must first dilute it because it is also cytotoxic

<u>Risks and Complications of Suturing Include:</u>

- Infections
- Abscess
- Damage to underlying tissue
- Scarring

Remember: Suturing is your LAST resort for wound closure and should only be done when medical help is delayed. If you ever have to suture another person it is important that the individual receives an evaluation by a physician as soon as possible.

Training

Do not underestimate the value of training when it comes to obtaining and maintaining medical skills. As with many skills you cannot have the mindset that you will train one time and never need to train again. Medical training requires a commitment on your part to attend refresher training or to upgrade your skills so that you can provide a higher level of care. Regular training will also build your confidence when having to use your skills during a real event. The more times you practice your skills, especially in a stressful training environment, the more likely you will be to perform well under the stress of an actual event. You owe it to the people that you treat to be well prepared as their life may literally be in your hands. If you make a mistake the patient may die due to your negligence. This is a mistake that you will have to live with for the rest of your life. Keep in mind that you can be held liable.

The American Red Cross offer basic classes in first aid and CPR. You can also obtain some very basic first aid training with your local Community Emergency Response Team (CERT.) Many local community colleges offer Emergency Medical Technology (EMT) classes which provide a solid foundation of rudimentary skills.

Good Samaritan Laws

According to the American Red Cross[xii]:

"All states have passed Good Samaritan laws or acts that give legal protection to lay rescuers who act in good faith with no expectation of remuneration and are not guilty of gross negligence or willful misconduct. The type of rescuer covered and the scope of protection vary from state to state."

When you are properly trained and act within the confines of your training everyone wins. Never provide care above your level of training such as using a nasopharyngeal airway or conducting a chest needle decompression when you have not received formal training in these procedures.

We live in a litigious society and you are likely to end up being sued if you perform care that you are not qualified to provide. In such cases Good Samaritan Laws will not offer you any protection. Even though your intentions might be in the right place you can find yourself in a very expensive predicament that was completely avoidable. Take the time to look up the law in the area that you live. This little bit of research may save you a lot of future problems.

Following are two examples of Good Samaritan Laws from Arizona and New York:

State of Arizona[xiii]:

32-1471. Health care provider and any other person; emergency aid; nonliability

Any health care provider licensed or certified to practice as such in this state or elsewhere, or a licensed ambulance attendant, driver or pilot as defined in section 41-1831, or any other person who renders emergency care at a public gathering or at the scene of an emergency occurrence gratuitously and in good faith shall not be liable for any civil or other damages as the result of any act or omission by such person rendering the emergency care, or as the result of any act or failure to act to provide or arrange for further medical treatment or care for the injured persons, unless such person, while rendering such emergency care, is guilty of gross negligence.

Building a Trauma Kit

State of New York^{xiv}

New York Good Samaritan Act

NYS Public Health Law, Article 30 - Emergency Medical Services; 3000-a.

Emergency medical treatment.

1. Except as provided in subdivision six of section six thousand six hundred eleven, subdivision two of section six thousand five hundred twenty-seven, subdivision one of section six thousand nine hundred nine and sections six thousand five hundred forty-seven and six thousand seven hundred thirty-seven of the education law, any person who voluntarily and without expectation of monetary compensation renders first aid or emergency treatment at the scene of an accident or other emergency outside a hospital, doctor's office or any other place having proper and necessary medical equipment, to a person who is unconscious, ill, or injured, shall not be liable for damages for injuries alleged to have been sustained by such person or for damages for the death of such person alleged to have occurred by reason of an act or omission in the rendering of such emergency treatment unless it is established that such injuries were or such death was caused by gross negligence on the part of such person. Nothing in this section shall be deemed or construed to relieve a licensed physician, dentist, nurse, physical therapist or registered physician's

assistant from liability for damages for injuries or death caused by an act or omission on the part of such person while rendering professional services in the normal and ordinary course of his or her practice.

2. A person who, or entity, partnership, corporation, firm or society that, purchases or makes available resuscitation equipment that facilitates first aid, as required by law or local law, shall not be liable for damages arising either from the use of that equipment by a person who voluntarily and without expectation of monetary compensation renders first aid or emergency treatment at the scene of an accident or medical emergency, or from the use of defectively manufactured equipment; provided that this subdivision shall not limit the person's or entity's, partnership's, corporation's, firm's or society's liability for his, her or its own negligence, gross negligence or intentional misconduct.

3013.

Immunity from liability.

1. Notwithstanding any inconsistent provision of any general, special or local law, a voluntary ambulance service or voluntary advanced life support first response service described in section three thousand one of this article and any member thereof who is a certified first responder, an emergency medical technician, an advanced emergency medical technician or a person acting under the direction of an

emergency medical technician or advanced emergency medical technician and who voluntarily and without the expectation of monetary compensation renders medical assistance in an emergency to a person who is unconscious, ill or injured shall not be liable for damages for injuries alleged to have been sustained by such person or for damages for the death of such person alleged to have occurred by reason of an act or omission in the rendering of such medical assistance in an emergency unless it is established that such injuries were or such death was caused by gross negligence on the part of such certified first responder, emergency medical technician or advanced emergency medical technician or person acting under the direction of an emergency medical technician or advanced emergency medical technician.

2. Nothing in this section shall be deemed to relieve any such voluntary ambulance service or voluntary advanced life support first response service from liability for damages or injuries or death caused by an act or omission on the part of any person other than a certified first responder, an emergency medical technician, advanced emergency medical technician or person acting under the direction of an emergency medical technician or advanced emergency medical technician acting in behalf of the voluntary ambulance service or voluntary advanced life support first response service.

3. Nothing in this section shall be deemed to relieve or alter the liability of any such voluntary ambulance service or members for damages or injuries or death arising out of the operation of motor vehicles.

4. A certified first responder, emergency medical technician or advanced emergency medical technician, whether or not he or she is acting on behalf of an ambulance service or advanced life support first response service, who voluntarily and without the expectation of monetary compensation renders medical assistance in an emergency to a person who is unconscious, ill or injured shall not be liable for damages alleged to have been sustained by such person or for damages for the death of such person alleged to have occurred by reason of an act or omission in the rendering of such medical assistance in an emergency unless it is established that such injuries were or such death was caused by gross negligence on the part of such certified first responder, emergency medical technician or advanced emergency medical technician.

5. Notwithstanding any inconsistent provision of any general, special or local law, any physician who voluntarily and without the expectation of monetary compensation provides indirect medical control, as defined in paragraph (b) of subdivision fifteen of section three thousand one of this article, to a voluntary ambulance service or voluntary advanced

life support first response service described in section three thousand one of this article shall not be liable for damages for injuries or death alleged to have been sustained by any person as a result of such medical direction unless it is established that such injuries or death were caused by gross negligence on the part of such physician.

As you can see the Good Samaritan Law in Arizona is much shorter and more concise than the law in New York. I strongly urge you to research the law in your state. If you do not understand the nuances of the law it would be a good idea to seek the advice of an attorney for clarification. Many states have their laws available for free online.

Good Samaritan Laws

It is your responsibility to know the Good Samaritan Laws that apply to you in order to minimize liability.

After the Trauma

You arrive at the scene of an accident before anyone else and you provide care at the level that you have been trained. Eventually, first responders will get on scene and take over patient care. Your role is now done. You provided the best care possible with the training that you have received and with the kit that you have designed. The care that you gave may save the person's life. At least that is the goal.

As you go about your day you begin to settle down. Your heart is no longer pounding and you are breathing normally. The adrenaline rush is gone. For a while you are amped up and then you feel like you need a nap. Dealing with a crisis can take its toll on you both physically and psychologically. It is important to remember to take care of yourself. Sometimes we focus so much on being prepared to help others that we forget to take care of ourselves. This is not healthy. It is also difficult to take care of others if you are not physically and mentally fit. This is true whether you are a first responder or a prepared and helpful citizen.

It is also important to understand that people may die despite your best efforts. Knowing that you provided the best possible care and did everything within your power to help the person may help you to accept the fact that people will die. Many times I would work with individuals who would become very emotional when they were unable to save a patient. Typically this individuals were the "trauma jocks" who only wanted the trauma calls. They end up bearing a huge burden over time. Yes, some emergencies will stick with us for the rest of our life. I'm sure people at the Boston Marathon bombing will never forget the carnage of dead bodies and lost limbs. The same for the terrorist attacks on 9/11. I still remember calls where people died that will probably remain with me until I am gone. It has taught me that life is precious. Time goes by fast and for some life is cut far too short. Bad things happen to good people. Sometimes we do not understand the reasoning for such darkness and loss.

Whether you are a prepper, law enforcement officer, firefighter, paramedic, banker, cook, or lawyer it is important to look after yourself. You may have made the decision to build a trauma kit to care for yourself, your family and others. Just remember that there are many outcomes that we do not have control over. Whether your profession is to help others or you rarely use your emergency skills it is important to have a support system that can help you through difficult times especially when the outcome is not what you sought.

For me building a trauma kit is an enjoyable process. It allows me to know that I am prepared for an emergency and that I have the knowledge, skills, and abilities to help others at the worst possible time. On the flip side I also realize that the time I help another person the truth is that their day is not going very well. When caring for another human being remember to always treat that person with respect and dignity.

Hopefully you will never need to use your trauma kit. But if you do it is comforting knowing that you have the skills and a quality kit to provide care. Life can be unpredictable so it is always good to be prepared.

Good luck and stay safe.

Summary

When designing your kit remember that you have the ability to change and modify the kit, over time, as necessary. You may find that some products do not meet your expectations or your kit is too large or small. Additionally, new products are constantly being developed based on research much of which is provided by the military. Current products are improved to be more effective and efficient. It is important to keep up on such changes by conducting research to find which components will suit your needs best. Know the pros and cons of each component in your kit and know how to use them under less than ideal circumstances. View your kit as a "dynamic" kit that changes over time rather than a "static" kit that becomes stagnant over time.

Regardless of which specific products you carry in your kit the one factor that cannot be overlooked is your training. ***You are the most important element in providing medical care.*** Receiving top quality initial training that is followed up on a regular basis with continuing education to improve your medical skills is a must. Medical skills are perishable and will degrade over time if you do not practice or use the skills. Quality training should include the use of scenarios that progressively incorporates increasing levels of stress and complexity. You need the knowledge, skills, and abilities to know what to do in a crisis to save lives. A severe hemorrhage can lead to death within a matter of minutes. Your ability to provide aid can mean the difference between life and death. You may have to perform care in an environment that is: cold, wet, dirty, dusty, hot, humid, blowing wind, low-light, etc. Sometimes you have to just *"embrace the suck."* The question you must ask yourself is:

Is my training preparing me for the worst case scenario?

If your answer is no, then you need to seek out better training. Remember, someone's life may depend on you!

Resources

- North American Rescue

    www.narescue.com/

- Rescue Essentials

    www.rescue-essentials.com/

- Adventure Medical Kits

    www.adventuremedicalkits.com/

- BLACKHAWK

    www.blackhawk.com/

- Eleven 10

    www.1110gear.com/

- Tactical Medical Packs

    www.tacticalmedicalpacks.com/

- HemCon

    www.hemcon.com/

- Z-Medica

    www.z-medica.com/index.asp

Building a Trauma Kit

- Voodoo Tactical

    www.voodootactical.net

- High Speed Gear

    www.highspeedgear.com/medical-pouches.html

- TierOne

    www.tierone.org

- Combat Application Tourniquet

    http://combattourniquet.com/

- Sam Medical Products

    www.sammedical.com/

- Rusch, Inc.

    www.ashermanchestseal.com/

- H&H Medical Corporation

    www.gohandh.com/

- Betadine

    www.betadine.com/

- Water-Jel

    www.waterjel.com/

- Laerdal Face Masks

    www.laerdal.com/us/

- Community Emergency Response Team

    www.fema.gov/community-emergency-response-teams

- American Red Cross Training

    www.redcross.org/what-we-do/training-education

Other Works by Gunner Morgan

1. Trauma Care for the Worst Case Scenario
2. Practical Defense for the Untrained Person
3. Psychology of Preppers: Mental Health Issues
4. Reality" in Reality Survival Shows

All are available on Amazon.

References

[i] World Report On Road Traffic Injury Prevention, http://www.who.int/violence_injury_prevention/publications/road_traffic/world_report/en/

[ii] U.S. Department of Health and Human Services, http://www.cdc.gov/nchs/data/hus/hus12.pdf

[iii] World Report on Child Injury Prevention, http://www.who.int/violence_injury_prevention/child/en/

[iv] http://ovc.ncjrs.gov/ncvrw2013/pdf/StatisticalOverviews.pdf

[v] Annual Disaster Statistical Review 2012: The numbers and trends, http://reliefweb.int/sites/reliefweb.int/files/resources/ADSR_2012.pdf

[vi] Civilian EMS Should Consider Tourniquets, http://www.jems.com/article/patient-care/civilian-ems-should-consider-tourniquets

[vii] Ibid

[viii] Prehospital topical hemostatic agents – A review of the current literature, PHTLS Executive Committee, Lance E. Stuke, M.D. MPH, http://www.naemt.org/Libraries/Trauma%20Resources/Prehospital%20Tobpical%20Hemostatic%20Agents.sflb

[ix] Ibid

[x] Butler, Frank. "Management of Open Pneumothorax in Tactical Combat Casualty Care: TCC Guidelines Change 13-02." Journal of Special Operations Medicine Volume 13, Edition 3/Fall 2013

[xi] http://www.waterjel.com/why-water-jel/

[xii] http://www.redcrosstrainingclasses.org/uploads/1/0/1/9/10191481/good_samaritan_laws.pdf

[xiii] http://www.azleg.gov/FormatDocument.asp?inDoc=/ars/32/01471.htm&Title=32&DocType=ARS

[xiv] http://www.slssdp.org/goodsam/New_York_Good_Samaritan_Act.pdf

www.ingramcontent.com/pod-product-compliance
Lightning Source LLC
Chambersburg PA
CBHW071755170526
45167CB00003B/1037